I0106532

RELAXING BY A WATERFALL

A meditative story to massage your body
and relax your mind

BOOKS IN THE NATUREBODY® SERIES

—

Walking in an Ancient Forest

Camping Under the Night Sky

Relaxing by a Waterfall

A Peaceful Winter Ski

Swimming in a Tropical Sea

A Healing Coastal Walk

Relaxing in the High Desert

A Spirited Mountain Hike

The complete
NatureBody® Connection
program is available at

www.aquaterramassage.com

A NATUREBODY® MASSAGE STORY

Relaxing by a
WATERFALL

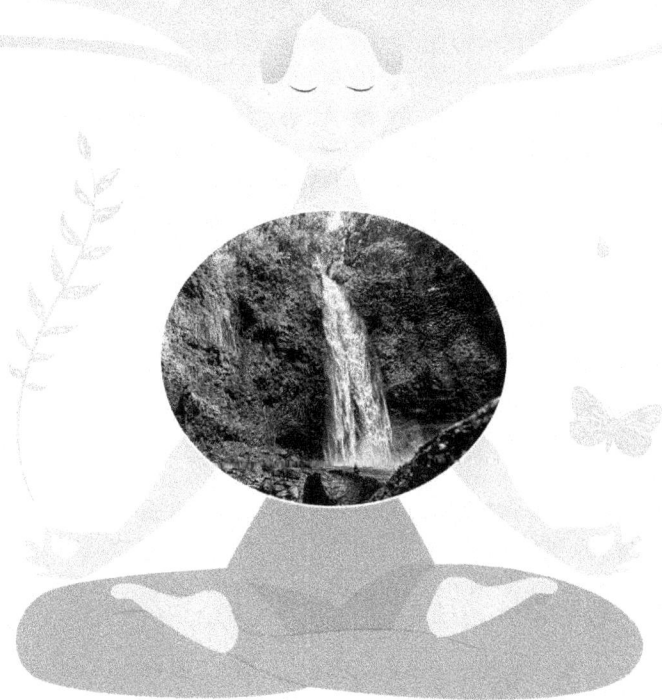

A meditative story to massage your body
and relax your mind

FAYE KRIPPNER *and* ERIK KRIPPNER

Disclaimer: This book does not offer medical advice to the reader and is not intended as a replacement for appropriate healthcare and treatment. For such advice, readers should consult a licensed physician.

Copyright © 2021 Erik Krippner, B.S., LMT, and Faye Krippner, B.A., LMT

All rights reserved. No portion of this book may be reproduced in any form without permission from the author or publisher, except as permitted by U.S. copyright law. For permissions contact info@aquaterramassage.com.

ISBN: 978-1-959772-06-4

Cover art provided by Envato Elements. Cover design by Faye Krippner and Erik Krippner.

Release Date for First Printed Edition 2023.

Media Inquiries: If you would like to contact the authors, please send an email to press@aquaterramassage.com.

Faye Krippner, B.A., LMT and Erik Krippner, B.S., LMT have been licensed by the Oregon Board of Massage Therapy since 2003. Oregon License Numbers: 10233 & 10234

Experience the entire NatureBody® Connection at
www.aquaterramassage.com

Dedicated to you

and your connection

to nature

along

your flow of life.

Index of Reflections

On Nature's Touch 6

On Flow 8

Breathing Length Into Your Spine 10

On Springy Legs 14

Sound's Influence on the Body 16

On the Healing Effects of Cool Water . . . 18

The Positive Effects of Negative Ions . . . 22

Hydrating Your Spine 24

On Connection 28

Contents

HOW TO USE THIS BOOK   IX

INTRODUCTION   1

THE HEADWATERS   5
Relaxation and Breathing

PILLARS OF STRENGTH   13
Leg Massage

A CASCADE OF RELIEF   21
Spinal Flow

TAKING THE PLUNGE   27
Full Body Relaxation

GRATITUDE   31
A Blessing From the Waterfall

ACKNOWLEDGMENTS   33

NOTES   35

JOURNAL   39

ABOUT THE AUTHORS   80

How to Use This Book

Humans have lived in balance with our bodies and the earth for 2.6 million years. Our bodies are designed for this planet. It is natural to walk on uneven ground, climb mountains, run long distances, swim, and most of all, to deeply breathe fresh air. Our wild planet heals and strengthens us by making us more flexible and fluid.

Your body is born of this earth. Earth is here to support you. Unfortunately, the stresses of life pull us off balance, and can leave us feeling physically sore and mentally anxious. This creative journey into relaxation is a way to remember your natural balance and create new muscle memories.

As massage therapists, we understand how a relaxed body feels: how it breathes, how it moves, how it is balanced in space. This NatureBody® massage story shares the full spectrum of massage: body, mind and spirit. Our intention is to empower you to find healing within yourself.

Visualization can have powerful effects on your body.[1] In this guided visualization, you will exercise your mind and imagination to deeply relax and bring your body back to center.

If you are injured or your ability to move is limited, then visualization is even more important! Studies have shown that when you imagine moving, the same areas of your brain activate as if you are actually moving those specific muscles.[2] Through visualization, you are virtually exercising your body.

We are intending for you to have a tangible, physical response to the ideas in this book. The power of this story lies in the vividness of your imagination. Read slowly. Pause. Use all of your senses to experience the story. Imagine the changes in humidity. Feel the gentle breeze on your skin. Hear the soothing sound of the wind. Smell the fresh scent of the life around you. Use your vibrant imagination to experience every detail in this story.

Put yourself in the story. Try to experience every sensation in your body. If you feel like moving, do it! Trust your instincts. Imagine what it feels like to move through the story: your muscles warming and stretching... your breathing deepening... your heartbeat slowing as you deeply relax. Let these sensations come to you at the speed of thought. This isn't about concentrating as much as it is about experiencing.

Each time you practice visualizing this story, your experience will become more vibrant. Your body is your wilderness to explore and understand. Your mind is your canvas for new muscle memories.

The Reflections are our personal notes to you. They offer you insight into some of the concepts in the story. Use them to spark your own creative thoughts about connection and healing.

The Notes section is full of wonderful articles and books that we have selected for you. If you feel interested in a topic, we highly recommend you look at the notes to explore the topic further.

The Journal at the end of the book gives you an opportunity to enhance and deepen your meditation. We have asked you a few thought-provoking questions to help you get started. Feel free to write or draw. Journal as creatively as you are inspired. This is your time to dream of the supportive connections between your body and nature.

There is much to discover about your relationship with your body and the beautiful world around you. Find a comfortable place to relax and enjoy. Prepare to be transported to a setting where you can unwind, immersed in nature, and experience the unbridled freedom of the wild!

From Wellness To Oneness,

Erik and Faye
Your Virtual Massage Therapists

FROM WELLNESS TO ONENESS

Wherever you are,

however you feel,

whatever your state of wellness,

know that

healing is at hand.

Your body is always seeking balance

and looking for opportunities to restore.

Through wellness,

may you come to oneness

with your body,

your mind,

your spirit,

and the beautiful Earth that supports us all.

Introduction

Water circulates around our planet and through our bodies. A cascading waterfall is one step in water's perpetual flow around the planet.

Spending time in and around a waterfall is a healing, full body experience. Waterfalls are energizing and blissfully peaceful. Whether we sit and watch a waterfall from a distance, or immerse ourselves in its flowing waters, we experience healing and renewal.

Waterfalls have many variations: from a stepped creek to a powerful torrent plunging hundreds of feet. We are soothed into meditation as we gaze at falling water. Our minds clear as we listen to the symphony of flowing water, from a light trickle to a booming, thunderous roar. Waterfalls have many personalities to suit our healing needs.

Let your stress flow away in this waterfall paradise as you strengthen your spirit with water, the elixir of life.

To experience the entire

NatureBody® Connection

scan this QR code

or go to

www.aquaterramassage.com / naturebodygift / waterfall

A gift for you, dear reader.

A special reading by the authors awaits you
at the link above.

CHAPTER ONE

The Headwaters

RELAXATION AND BREATHING

The trees cast a pleasant shade through the serene forest. Small mountain wildflowers edge the narrow footpath I have been traveling. Hiking down from the mountaintop, I begin to smell water in the air.

My walk through this peaceful forest has led me to a shallow stream. I stroll next to the quietly chattering water as it flows among mossy, old-growth trees. The forest glows with a healing green hue. Diffuse sunlight refracts through the leaves, lighting the living greenery like stained glass. The scent of the forest fills the humid air in this natural cathedral.

I feel at home here.
My breathing is slow.
My heartbeat is calm.

On Nature's Touch

*"I imagine their circular movement
like fingertips massaging my temples."*

The textures and movements of nature can inspire your
own healing touch.

Place your fingertips on your temples. Lightly circle your
temples with the gentleness of a breeze moving the fronds
of small ferns. Feel the muscles of your face and scalp
changing as you relax under your own touch.

Water glides smoothly over rounded stones in the stream
like a soft hand gliding across your skin. Place your hand
on your forearm. Let your hand conform to the shape of
your arm. Keeping your hand soft like water over stone,
stroke upward toward your heart, returning the venous
streams of circulation to your center.

The feathery moss on the bank of the creek invites you to
take off your shoes and explore the natural sensitivity of
your feet. As you wiggle and spread your toes, the muscles
of your feet stretch and strengthen. Your arches flex and
release to conform to the textures of the earth. There are
over 14,000 nerve endings in your feet, helping to
interpret the weight of the world as you know it. Feel the
sensitivity of your feet as you brush them across the floor.

You are developing a sensitive touch. The textures of
nature are teaching you to restore and heal.

A log lies next to the little stream. It looks like a lovely place to rest. I sit on the mossy log and watch the creek dance and swirl. The clear water looks refreshing.

I take off my shoes and wade into the shallow water. A short distance downstream, the creek disappears from view. I am standing in the safety of the forest at the headwaters of a lively waterfall.

Breezy updrafts carry vapor from the falling water, gently sprinkling my face with cool mist. My eyes are drawn to the magnificent view across the verdant river valley to the mountains in the distance.

I close my eyes and imagine the waterfall below. I anticipate the tranquil energy of this creek coming to life as the water falls. Like a flexed muscle, the stream's energy is expressed as it falls and will relax upon its return to tranquil waters.

> *This peaceful stream will briefly flex its strength*
> > *through the power of falling water*
> > *and then relax to its quiet flow.*

> *Its power and peace will join the great river,*
> > *and as with all great rivers,*
> > *flow toward,*
> > *and be united in the ocean.*

I return to the fallen log next to the stream. The creek is crystal clear. Rocks of many colors marble the stream bed. Water glides smoothly over the rounded stones. Small ferns cling to the stream side, gently waving in the breeze.

> *I imagine their circular movement*
> > *like fingertips massaging my temples.*

On Flow

> *"The sense of flow soothes my spine and cleanses my spirit."*

Air and water continually flow across the planet, mingling and separating in a perpetual dance. Clouds form, change, and dissipate as they travel across the sky. Ocean waves cast a misty veil into the air. Fog condenses over a lake on a cool morning. The spinning of the earth adds a swirl of movement to the weather systems.[3]

As you breathe, imagine the flow of air and water spiraling in your own body. Feel the air spin in your sinuses as you inhale, moistening and warming in your nose and throat. Draw your inhale into your body. Invite it deep into your lungs.

Your deepest breaths will feel like they fill your whole torso all the way down into your hips. Imagine your breath pooling in your pelvis, like a calm lake. Allow a sense of buoyancy to rise up and expand the soft spaces between your bones.

When you exhale, picture the air flowing upwards as if an underground artesian spring is forcing water up to the surface from the pressure below. Squeeze your abs lightly to exhale more completely. Your humid exhale reunites with the moisture of the atmosphere.

Breathing joins you with the flow of life, connecting you to all that is around you. Your breath feeds your energy, stokes your inner fire, and brings life to your tissues. Your living essence fills the universe.

The creek is nestled in this peaceful forest, and I am put at ease as I watch it.

> I wriggle my toes
>> in the soft, feathery moss
>> edging the creek.

> My breathing slows.

> I picture my breath
>> sinking down into my lower belly,
>> like a pool of still water
>> within me.

> The pool grows deeper
>> as my breath sinks down
>> to the base of my pelvis,
>> spreading my sitting bones.

> My lower belly expands softly
>> as I breathe in.

> My exhale's grounding energy
>> sinks down to my feet,
>> and into the moss.

> As my breath feels lower and lower in my body,
>> my shoulders drop.
>> My chest relaxes.

Breathing Length Into Your Spine

"My spine lengthens as I engage my abdominal muscles..."

Your abdominal and back muscles naturally work together to hold you upright against the pull of gravity. In order for your spine to feel relaxed and healthy, you need muscle tone throughout your core and around your trunk: in the front, sides, and back of your body.

When your posture is balanced and your abs toned, the muscles around your torso share the effort of holding you upright. Simply tightening your abdominal muscles supports your spine, takes the pressure off your vertebrae, and eases the effort of your back muscles.

Try this exercise. Squeeze your abdominal muscles gently, and picture them hugging your spine. Tighten them as if you are drawing your belly button in and up. Next, breathe low into your pelvis to grow taller. Reach out of the crown of your head while grounding through your feet, as if your spine is lengthening in both directions. This exercise uses your breath to bring more strength and flexibility to your spine. Each breath renews strength and encourages space between your bones.

Joseph Pilates said, "You are only as young as your spine is flexible." With a free and flexible spine, you are able to enjoy the activities that keep you feeling vibrant and alive.

I passively allow my breath to fill me
    like a waterfall
    cascading through my body
    and out my feet.

The sense of flow
    soothes my spine and cleanses my spirit.

Deep relaxation settles into my being.

I lean back slightly, balancing my upper body on my hips.

My spine lengthens
    as I engage my abdominal muscles
    and draw them upward from my balanced pelvis.

I grow taller.
    My vertebrae lengthen away from one another,
    allowing the fluid in, around,
    and between my vertebrae to flow,
    like my own internal cascade.

My shoulders drop.
    My arms feel heavy, and my hands, relaxed.
    I can feel the energy of the stream
    coursing through my veins.

I open my vision to the edges of my eyes,
    and take in all that is around me.

I am aware of the wind waving in the trees above and the water flowing around my feet. Time seems to slow.

CHAPTER TWO

Pillars of Strength

LEG MASSAGE

Sunlight streams through the trees, dancing on the forest floor. Birdsong is accompanied by the whisper of trees, musically playing the strings of wind.

A small bird alights on the log next to me. Just as quickly, it flitters to a nearby branch, cocking its head toward the stream. Its staccato movements seem rehearsed as it flutters from perch to perch to gain perspective. It inspires me to move and see the waterfall from a new perspective.

I resume my walk to the bottom of the falls. The path winds away from the stream, gradually descending along the contours of the mountain.

On Springy Legs

"My strong leg muscles wrap around bone and support my joints. Like the coils of a spring, my active muscles cushion my descent."

Even though walking downhill feels like it should be easy, it can be quite hard on the body. It seems easy to "fall" downhill, landing heavily on our feet with each step. However, what "feels" easy is not the best for our bodies.

Our knees and shins can get very sore when walking downhill. The impact of each step sends shockwaves through our joints.

When you walk downhill, keep yourself tall and upright. Bend your knees and reach for your next step. Pull your front leg back strongly. Even if you feel tired, keep your legs engaged and knees bent. That will take the pounding impact out of your stride and protect your joints.

The key to cushioning our joints is to keep our leg muscles active. Our muscles absorb the impact of walking and minimize the jarring shock of our steps. Our legs become more like coiled springs and we move more smoothly.

Done with intention, walking downhill can be fun and exhilarating. When you use good form, you feel like you are gliding smoothly downhill. With strong, powerful legs you can enjoy the feeling of a fluid stride.

I appreciate the challenge of walking downhill,
   keeping my hips balanced over my feet.

I bend my knees
   to cushion my joints
   with my powerful leg muscles.

I walk tall and upright.

My strong leg muscles wrap around bone
   and support my joints.

Like the coils of a spring,
   my active muscles
   cushion my descent.

The forest canopy seems far above me now. I am making good progress downhill, and keep my smooth pace.

Sound's Influence on the Body

"Its music reverberates through my body."

The sounds of nature relax and soothe our nervous system. Listening to nature's soundscape can brighten your mood, help your cognitive focus, and inspire creativity. Nature sounds are healing for the body, both alleviating pain and improving sleep.[4]

The varied frequencies of a waterfall allow you to deepen your listening experience. Imagine you are standing next to a waterfall. Listen to the sounds of falling water. Visualize how each frequency vibrates within your body.

Feel the booming presence of the falls. The thunderous water vibrates through your center, awakening your senses to your core.

Deep-throated rumbles speak deeply to your bones and muscles like the penetrating effect of a deep tissue massage.

The frothy, effervescent hiss can feel like it tingles your scalp. Let the whispers of mist send shivers through your head and neck.

The musical flow of water delights your skin and soothes your senses. A waterfall's chorus sings to your body. Its symphonic power dissolves your excess tension and improves your sense of well being.

At the bottom of the hill, the trail winds back to the creek. The waterfall's distant hush becomes louder, until its booming presence dominates the soundscape.

> *The waterfall is a symphony of sound,*
>   *from its frothy, effervescent hiss*
>   *to its deep-throated rumbles.*

> *Its music reverberates through my body.*

Towering walls of black rock contain the scene of the waterfall. Columnar basalt was once fluid lava that cooled into perfectly square columns of even width and varying lengths. Water flows beautifully down and around these geometric shapes.

> *The rigidity of rock contrasts to the fluidity of water.*

The rock wall parts the water into a series of smaller cascades, all plunging into a deep, clear pool. Water sheens on the rock next to me. I admire the ferns and flowers that grow in its cracks. Hanging mosses are adorned with silvery sequins of water droplets.

> *Sun streams through the mist of the falls,*
>   *refracting rainbows*
>   *in the air around me.*

On the Healing Effects of Cool Water

"The contrast of the cool water and warm sun sends circulation rushing through my veins."

Cool water contrasts with the heat of our warm-blooded bodies, and can be very healing. When we immerse in cold water, our capillaries constrict, squeezing fluid out of the cooled area. As our bodies warm again, our blood vessels dilate, bringing fresh, nutrient-rich fluid into the area.[5] The constriction of cold and the dilation of heat creates a pumping effect that cleanses and nourishes our tissues.

Our bodies respond well to therapeutic variations in temperatures. Cool water can relieve our sore muscles by decreasing inflammation. Taking cold showers has been shown to increase endorphins, boost our energy levels, and stimulate our immune system.[6]

Any temperature lower than your internal body temperature will have some effect on your circulation. Start comfortably, and gradually work your way toward cooler temperatures.

Temperature ranges of water

Cold water:	55° to 65° F	13°-18° C
Cool water:	66° to 80° F	19°-26° C
Tepid water:	81° to 92° F	27°-33° C
Warm water:	93° to 97° F	34°-36° C
Hot water:	98° to 104° F	37°-40° C

On this warm day,
 the cool, misty spray
 from the falls
 is welcome on my skin.

My pores tighten in the cool spray.

The contrast of the cool water and warm sun
 sends circulation rushing through my veins.

I feel invigorated.

CHAPTER THREE

A Cascade of Relief

SPINAL FLOW

A side trail leads behind the waterfall. I walk behind the curtain of water and find a protected rock shelter: tall enough for me to stand in, deep enough to be away from the falls. The walls of this cavern are moist from the atomized air, yet I am protected from the heavy spray.

Over the years, churning water has scoured out the exposed rock that used to exist here, creating a space behind the waterfall. The persistent power of water has broken the rocks and carried them away, creating this shelter. Looking out through the flat cascade, I admire the surging texture of the water. Back here, the sound of the falls echoes. I can hear the percussion in the symphonic fall of water.

Small birds find shelter behind waterfalls, building nests in cracks in the wall. Birds can fly sideways through falling water, parting the cascade with one wing while then sliding

The Positive Effects of Negative Ions

"I inhale, feeling the satisfying and rejuvenating effects of the healing mist."

Crashing water creates a swirl of cleansing air around it. We get a burst of uplifting energy by a waterfall.

As water plunges downward, water molecules collide, breaking molecular bonds. This releases negative ions into the air. Simply breathing this richly ionized, cleansing air is healing in many ways. Breathing negative ions can replenish our energy, enliven our mood, regulate our sleep, and help us think more clearly.[8]

You can enjoy richly ionized air in nature. Ionized air is created around a waterfall, in a rainstorm, at the ocean, and even in the shower. Breathe and allow your body to be permeated and refreshed with negative ions.

Enjoy your time in and around falling water, breathing the atmosphere that helps you feel invigorated.

their body underneath it.[7] They raise their young in the protection of the falls.

The crashing of the water ionizes the air.

I inhale,
    feeling the satisfying and rejuvenating effects
    of the healing mist.

When I exhale,
    I cleanse my body of stagnant energy.

My skin is damp.

I feel cleansed and joyful.

I walk back out from behind the falls and am greeted by the vibrant green hills that surround this clear pool. Birds flutter in the trees, and yellow butterflies float through the sunshine over the shimmering pool.

At the edge of the pool, a small cascade showers the rocks. I am drawn to its soft, effervescent water. I walk toward it and put my hand in the stream. Its tingling, frothy bubbles feel wonderful on my skin.

I stand under the cascade and feel it drumming on my shoulders and back.

My muscles soften under the beating of the water.

The constant downward rush
    soothes my muscles.

My neck and shoulders feel wonderfully open.

Hydrating Your Spine

"I imagine my midline narrowing and reaching,
like a fish migrating upstream."

Imagine you are a salmon, swimming up a waterfall. As you wriggle and narrow your body upward, you can feel your abdominal muscles engage. You are encouraging your spine to lengthen to its full height, taking pressure off the soft discs between your vertebrae.

A healthy abdomen is both strong and supple. Visualize swimming upstream, your spine stretching as you reach upward. A toned core supports your posture and frees your spine to be more flexible.

Rise tall out of your hips. Squeeze your abdomen to narrow your lower ribcage. Let your shoulders release down your back. Reach out of the crown of your head. Tuck your chin slightly. Soften your throat. Stretch your neck long. Breathe, and enjoy the feeling of your supple, dynamic spine.

Many of us think we need to do crunches to build our abdomen... we seek the elusive "six-pack" to know that we are strong and healthy. Many yogis warn against over-tightening our ab muscles,[9] instead encouraging a strong and supple abdomen that expands with your inhale and narrows with your exhale. Pilates workouts teach core strength to help you support your spine and stand taller.[10] You can free your spine with the strength of your core.

The muscles of my back cascade down my spine.

My muscles relax as the pulsing water
  blankets down my body,
    while my bones stand tall against the flow.

I tighten my abs to find more length in my lumbar spine.

I imagine my midline narrowing and reaching,
    like a fish migrating upstream.

While the water pounds my muscles
    down into buttery relaxation,
    my spine defies gravity
    and becomes more buoyant and supple.

My breath moves freely through my body.

I imagine myself becoming more fluid.

The water steadily smoothes the edges of rock,
    and soothes the edges of my tension.

A waterfall breaks apart the minerals of the earth and
carries them out to sea, nourishing all life along its path.
Likewise, this cascade is healing me, breaking apart my
tension and washing it away.

I feel nurtured and nourished in the flow,
    revived to support life along my path.

CHAPTER FOUR

Taking the Plunge

FULL BODY RELAXATION

I step forward out of the cascade and let the sun warm my skin. The pool of clear water in front of me looks deep and refreshing. It is irresistible.

I walk into the cool water until my body is submerged.

I relish the rush of coolness
and welcome the freedom of weightlessness as I float.

My joints feel joyous
as they surrender their strain from gravity.

I move my body like a seal through the water,
twisting and contorting,
reveling in the freedom of motion.

On Connection

"The flow of water connects us all."

Nature, our original home, provides our bodies the sustenance to live fully. It offers us emotional solace by showing us how things grow and live together in this changing world. Spending time in nature inspires us to be ourselves.

Water is nature's vital essence: the elixir of life. Water teaches us to flow. It is a catalyst for change. Water connects the land, the atmosphere, and all life. Its vapor swirls in clouds above. It flows down mountains, nourishes the land, and circulates through the ocean's deepest currents. It pools in aquifers deep underground. The water you drink has been flowing around the planet for millennia.[11]

Our bodies are over 50% water. It nourishes our cells. It lubricates our joints and cleanses our bodies. Water even helps conduct the electricity of thought.[12] Water flows in us and through us. We drink water. We expel water. We are continually exchanging water with the world around us. All life shares the need for water.

Like water, you are intimately connected to the living world. You are a part of the intricate web of all life.

I kick my way to the bottom of the pool. The rocks at the bottom are round and smooth. The rippling surface of the water refracts light, marbling the underwater world.

I surface and swim closer to the falls. The cascade creates an underwater dance of bubbles as it plunges into the pool. The water splashes around me and I squint and smile as I swim by. I flip over onto my back and look up at the falls.

> *The water is supporting me as I float.*
> > *I feel weightless.*
> > *My arms and legs bob*
> > *in the gentle rocking of the stream.*

> *I am immersed*
> > *in the sensation and sound of water.*

> *I breathe the atomized air.*
> > *I hear the pounding waterfall.*
> > *I feel the soft, fluid support of water.*

> *My body and mind are one in this idyllic setting.*

My mind is renewed in the mist of the waterfall. I have been given a refreshed perspective.

My body is relaxed from my time at the waterfall.
I feel prepared for what is to come.

> *I am connected to the stream,*
> > *on this step of its journey to the ocean.*

> *The flow of water connects us all.*[13]

CHAPTER FIVE

Gratitude

A BLESSING FROM THE WATERFALL

T hank you for this time by the waterfall.
Until we meet again,

*May the pounding of water
dissolve tension in your tissues.*

*May the negative ions of crashing water
positively refresh your outlook on life.*

May tranquil waters buoy and support you.

*May flowing water remind you of your connection
to all that is, and all that will be.*

Float on, Tranquil Wanderer.

Acknowledgments

Sandra Jeanne Franklin's lively spirit inspired us to live in the now. Thank you for showing us your delight in waterfalls. You jumped in every time.

We thoroughly enjoyed the BBC documentary, *Nature's Most Amazing Events*, for demonstrating how the flow of water nurtures the continuity of all life on this planet.

Thank you, Marty Ryan, for showing us how to "love our guts" and speak kindly to our bodies. Your teachings on abdominal massage deepened our appreciation for the buoyancy and flow of our internal organs.

Our fellow massage therapist, Jay Alvaro, has a talent at drumming that brings the percussive massage strokes of tapotement to life. His adept massage brings the power of a waterfall to the massage table.

Joseph Pilates' teachings emphasized the importance of core strength. Pilates taught us that there is so much more to strengthening our core than doing crunches. It teaches us to support our whole structure and improve our posture through abdominal strength. Thank you Teresa Lee, Fanina Padykula, Matt Lueders and Jessica Talisman for being our mentors in our pursuit of core strength.

ACKNOWLEDGMENTS

Notes

1. "What is Imagery?" *Johns Hopkins Medicine*, 2003, www.hopkinsmedicine.org/health/wellness-and-prevention/imagery.

2. Lohr, Jim. "Can Visualizing Your Body Doing Something Help You Learn to Do It Better?" *Scientific American*, 1 May 2015, www.scientificamerican.com/article/can-visualizing-your-body-doing-something-help-you-learn-to-do-it-better.

3. "The Coriolis Effect: Earth's Rotation and Its Effect on Weather." *National Geographic*, education.nationalgeographic.org/resource/coriolis-effect. Accessed on 17 January 2023.

4. Pena, Claudicet. "10 Years of Research Reveals That Listening To Nature Can Improve Your Overall Health." *My Modern Net*, 4 May 2021, mymodernmet.com/nature-sounds-health-study.

5. Mooventhan, A., & Nivethitha, L. "Scientific Evidence-Based Effects of Hydrotherapy on Various Systems of the Body." *North American Journal of Medical Sciences,* vol. 6, no. 5, 2016, pp. 199–209, doi.org/10.4103/1947-2714.132935.

6. Watson, Kathryn. "Cold Shower Benefits for Your Health." *Healthline,* 24 April 2017, www.healthline.com/health/cold-shower-benefits.

7. Funnell, Rachel. "Incredible Video Shows How Hummingbirds Shimmy Their Way Through Waterfalls." *IFLScience,* 19 August 2020, www.iflscience.com/incredible-video-shows-how-hummingbirds-shimmy-their-way-through-waterfalls-57040.

8. Hu, Y. Q., Niu, T. T., Xu, J. M., Peng, L., Sun, Q. H., Huang, Y., Zhou, J., & Ding, Y. Q. "Negative Air Ion Exposure Ameliorates Depression-Like Behaviors Induced by Chronic Mild Stress in Mice." *Environmental Science and Pollution Research International,* vol. 29, no. 41, 2022, pp. 62626–62636. doi.org/10.1007/s11356-022-20144-x.

9. "Forget Six-Pack Abs: What It Really Means to Have Strong Abdominals" *Yoga Journal,* 28 August 2007, www.yogajournal.com/teach/anatomy-yoga-practice/forget-six-pack-abs.

10. Finnie, Donna. "Does Pilates Make You Taller? What the Science Knows." *Pilates Moves You,* pilatesmovesyou.com/does-pilates-make-you-taller-what-the-science-knows. Accessed 17 January 2023.

11. "How Old is the Water We Drink?" *Discover Magazine,* 20 December 2022, www.discovermagazine.com/the-sciences/how-old-is-the-water-we-drink.

12. Gowin, Joshua. "Why Your Brain Needs Water." *Psychology Today*, 15 October 2010, www.psychologytoday.com/us/blog/you-illuminated/201010/why-your-brain-needs-water.

13. "The Natural Water Cycle" *United States Geologic Survey*, 2019, www.usgs.gov/media/images/natural-water-cycle-jpg.

NOTES

MEDITATION

Journal

This journal gives you a place to reflect on your experience as you read and meditate. With every meditation, your library of personal affirmations can grow. Some thoughts you might want to record, in words or drawings, are:

What were your favorite phrases or ideas in the story?

Describe the waterfall you visualized. What feelings did you notice as you traveled through your waterfall paradise? What physical sensations did you feel in your body as you read the story?

What is your relationship with water? What are your favorite ways to enjoy water (...sustenance, pleasure, sport)?

Write about connection, family, and flow. Describe the people, thoughts, memories, and ideas that give you a sense of belonging.

"I OPEN MY VISION TO THE
EDGES OF MY EYES, AND TAKE IN
ALL THAT IS AROUND ME."

MEDITATION

Try softening your focus by becoming aware of your entire field of vision. See the world all around you. Notice how much broader your awareness can be, and how much subtle movement you can see.

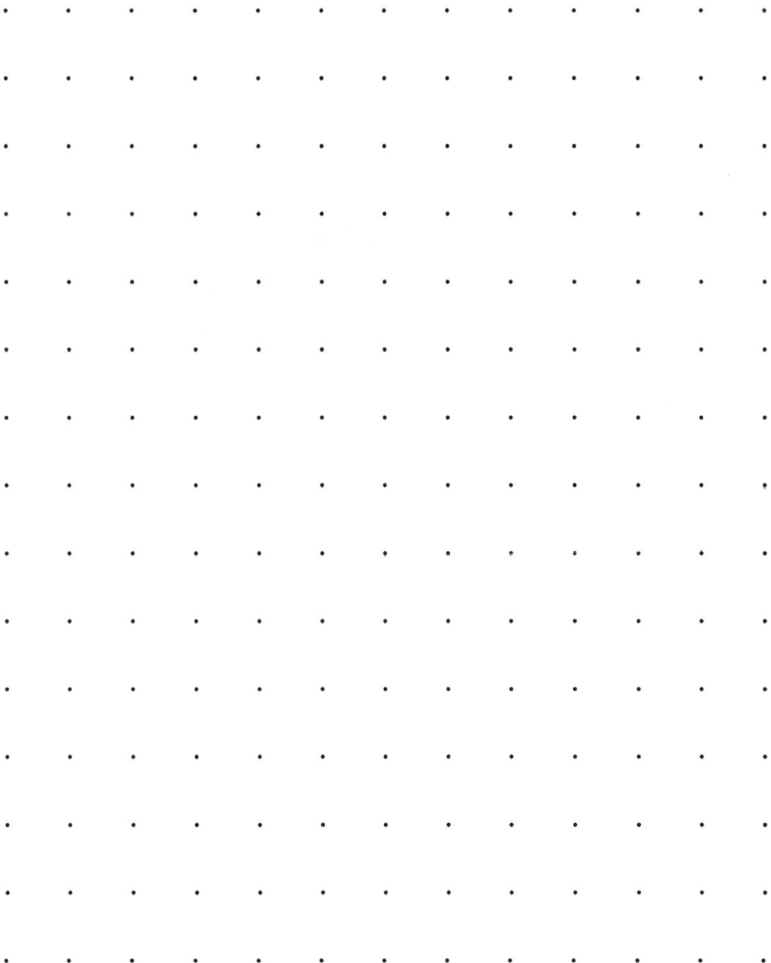

~

"BREEZY UPDRAFTS CARRY
VAPOR FROM THE FALLING
WATER, GENTLY SPRINKLING MY
FACE WITH COOL MIST."

MEDITATION

Nature can elicit many feelings within us: tranquility, inspiration, excitement, and joy. Where do you feel most uplifted and energized in nature? Can you sense how nature is renewing your being?

~

May the

pounding of water

DISSOLVE

TENSION

in your tissues.

"I PICTURE MY BREATH
SINKING DOWN INTO MY LOWER
BELLY, LIKE A POOL OF STILL WATER
WITHIN ME."

MEDITATION

Even when things feel tense and anxious, you can tap into your own inner reservoir of serenity. Your breath helps you connect with that tranquil place within you. Slow the pace of your breathing and become aware of your center. Feel your body and mind calm.

~

"THE FLOW OF WATER
CONNECTS US ALL."

Consider the many ways you use water. Where has this water come from? Where is it going? Water infuses every cell of your body. Since life began, water has been present in the clouds, the oceans, inside living cells, and is even permeates rock. Water connects you to all that has been, all that is, and all that will be.

~

May the

negative ions

of crashing water

POSITIVELY

REFRESH

your outlook on life.

"I STAND UNDER THE WATERFALL
AND FEEL IT POUND ON MY
SHOULDERS AND BACK."

MEDITATION

Sometimes gravity can be delivered in just the right way to help you release the weight of the world. Nature offers us many ways to receive relaxation. Our bodies respond to nature's stimuli. Where is your favorite place to relax in nature?

~

"THE PEACEFUL STREAM BRIEFLY SHOWS US ITS STRENGTH THROUGH THE POWER OF FALLING WATER AND THEN RETURNS TO TRANQUILITY BELOW."

MEDITATION

We all go through times where we have to be "on." We have to ride the wave and be strong. We must perform when we are needed.

Once that time has passed, you can return to a more peaceful rhythm.

Massage and meditation bring you back to your relaxed, healing center. When you connect to that serene place within you, you build an inner resilience to the stressors of life. You fortify your ability to relax.

~

May

tranquil waters

BUOY

and

SUPPORT

you.

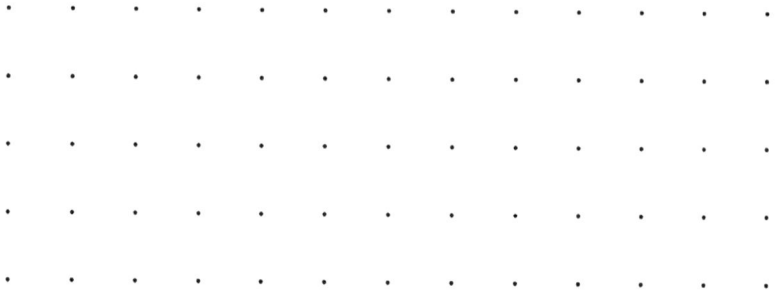

"COLUMNAR BASALT WAS ONCE
FLUID LAVA THAT COOLED INTO
PERFECTLY SQUARE COLUMNS...
WATER FLOWS BEAUTIFULLY DOWN
AND AROUND THESE GEOMETRIC
SHAPES."

MEDITATION

Our bodies shift and change through the day, through the seasons, and through our lifetimes. There is beauty and purpose to our ever-changing selves. A majestic mountain range was once fluid lava. Appreciate your evolving form, and the gifts that your body has to offer you.

~

"LOOKING OUT THROUGH THE
FLAT CASCADE, I ADMIRE THE
SURGING TEXTURE OF WATER."

MEDITATION

Picture yourself behind the sheeting stream of a waterfall. The cool, atomized air dampens your face. Focus on the falling water. Allow it to soothe you into a meditative sense of tranquility.

~

May

flowing water

remind you

of your

CONNECTION

to all

that is,

and all

that will be.

"I AM AWARE OF THE WIND WAVING
IN THE TREES ABOVE AND THE
WATER FLOWING AROUND MY FEET.
TIME SEEMS TO SLOW."

MEDITATION

It has been said that time flies when we are having fun. And yet, a dreamy day in nature, unencumbered by distractions, can feel like it lasts forever. When we bring ourselves fully into the moment, we enter nature's time.

~

"MY BREATHING SLOWS AND MY HEARTBEAT CALMS IN THIS NATURAL CATHEDRAL."

MEDITATION

Where do you feel the most comfortable? Close your eyes and mentally transport yourself to that place. Fully immerse yourself in your imagination. Notice the scents, textures, sights, and sounds in your peaceful refuge. As you experience this safe and comfortable setting, feel your body relax and your breathing slow. You are bringing yourself into a place of peace: experiencing a moment of serenity.

~

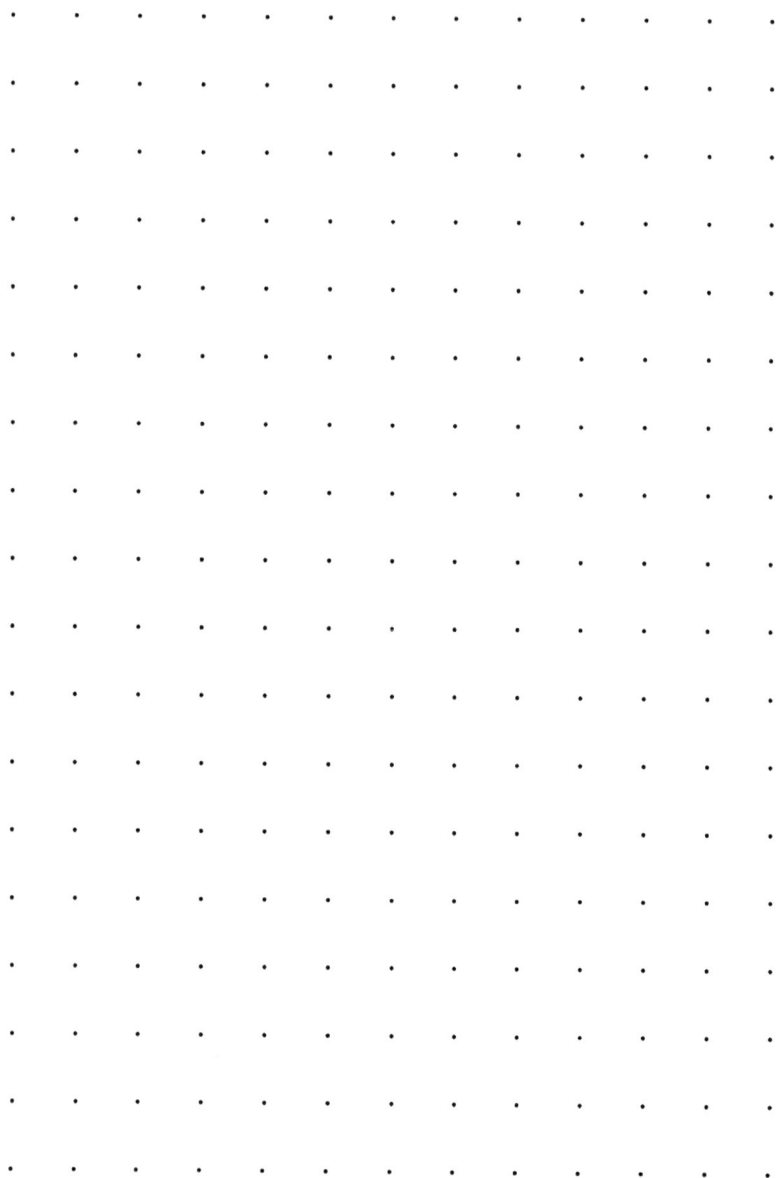

BLESSING
FROM THE WATERFALL

May the
pounding of water

DISSOLVE TENSION

in your tissues.

May the negative ions
of crashing water

POSITIVELY REFRESH

your outlook on life.

May
tranquil waters

BUOY AND SUPPORT

you.

May flowing water
remind you
of your

CONNECTION

to all that is,
and all
that will be.

About the Authors

Born and raised in New Orleans, Erik Krippner grew up with a po'boy in his hand and a song in his heart. As a boy, he spent his summers swimming, hiking, fishing, and sailing. After becoming an Eagle Scout, Erik dreamed of answering the call to "Go West, young man." He earned a Bachelor of Science degree in Forestry from Louisiana State University. Following his passion for adventure, Erik found his way to the mountains of the Pacific Northwest, his home to this day. After working in the forests of Oregon, Washington, Idaho, Alaska, Georgia, and Louisiana, Erik decided to focus his love of natural sciences on the study of human body through massage therapy.

Faye grew up in Oregon surrounded by family and old growth coastal forests. She spent many childhood weekends cross-country skiing, hunting for mushrooms, exploring coastal tide pools, and searching for crawdads in the Siuslaw River. Her love of books deepened when she became the editor of her high school and college's literary journals. Upon earning her Bachelor of Arts degree in Mathematics with honors from the Robert D. Clark Honors College at the University of Oregon, Faye became a technical writer and web developer. The whisper of a deeper purpose ignited her to study massage, where she met Erik.

Erik and Faye became friends in massage school at the East West College of the Healing Arts, in Portland, Oregon. In 2003, they founded Aqua Terra Massage, a therapeutic massage studio for friends and couples. Since then, they have practiced therapeutic massage together, side by side. They have spent years immersed in the study of massage, serving thousands of clients.

Faye and Erik have spent years exploring and writing about our beautiful world. They have sailed the blue waters of Fiji's Koro Sea, kayaked New Zealand's Marlborough Sound, and stargazed among the giraffes and elephants in Botswana. They have hiked the Appalachian Trail and paddled the tidally-influenced Columbia River in the Pacific Northwest. They have seen orca whales swim right under their kayaks, locked eyes with wild lions, and played hide-and-seek with an octopus. They have hiked thousands of miles together, kayaked and sailed hundreds, and spent countless evenings camping under the stars.

With a commitment to bringing more love and kindness
to this beautiful world, we offer this book to you.

www.aquaterramassage.com

www.ingramcontent.com/pod-product-compliance
Lightning Source LLC
Chambersburg PA
CBHW060254030426

42335CB00014B/1687